STOP Pain:
Steps to Self-empowerment

Dr. Bob Peddicord,
Clinical Psychologist

2/21/2023

Introduction

Pain often interferes with life and happiness. Steps provided here engage your inner strength and the natural power of your body to stop pain.

Medication may be added to supplement these steps for severe or persistent pain. However, narcotic based medication should be used very sparingly in order to avoid addiction, which can be very difficult to deal with.

When the steps of **STOP Pain** are combined with medication they can reduce both the amount of medication needed and the risk of addiction.

The steps of **STOP Pain** can also be used to stop anxiety and frustration. In addition, they can reduce fear and other painful emotions.

Copyright© 2017 & 2023

by Robert S. Peddicord, PhD;
All Rights Reserved.

No part of this publication may be reproduced, stored in a retrieval system, or transmitted, in any form or by any means, electronic, mechanical, photocopying, recording, or otherwise, without prior written permission from the author.

Unauthorized duplication of this material in any form is strictly prohibited.

ISBN: 9798813864506

Contents

Cautionary Note!	3
How Pain Works	4
How I Fell Asleep at the Dentist	6
Steps to **STOP** Pain	9
Practice the Steps of **STOP** Pain	17
Use Medication Cautiously	19
Combining **STOP** Pain with Medication	21
Comparing Medication & **STOP**	22
STOP to Go to Sleep at Night	32
Use on Phones & Tablets	34
About the Author	35

Cautionary Note!

Pain can let you know that medical attention is needed to explore underlying causes.

Pain may also let you know that you need to take a break so that you don't hurt yourself.

Once you have checked out a pain and decide that it is safe to proceed, you may use the steps in this manual to STOP the pain.

Endorsement

As a doctor practicing in an interventional pain medicine office, I have found Dr. Bob's **STOP** Pain book an excellent resource for patients. His book is straightforward and easy to follow and learn. His quick cue steps can be used in other situations too. I use them and recommend them.

Ben Zolper, M.D.; Anesthesiologist

How Pain Works

1. If you focus the your attention on pain, it will increase the pain.

2. Tensing up also increases pain!

3. Fear of pain empowers pain and makes it grow!

To STOP Pain,

it's important to relax and

turn your attention away

from pain,

thereby empower yourself.

How I Fell Asleep at the Dentist
By Dr. Bob Peddicord

Several years ago, a dentist was grinding on a broken tooth. It sounded like a jackhammer going off in my head and was driving me crazy. So, I decided to go away in my mind. First, I breathed slowly. Next, I tuned out and pictured a peaceful scene of a horse standing under a tree. A breeze was blowing through the horses tail and mane. The image was so vivid that I could imagine the breeze blowing across the hair on my arm. Then, I imagined the sound of pleasant music. Finally, I told myself: "I'm going to relax and be calm." The next thing I knew, the dental assistant asked the dentist whether I was OK, because I was snoring.

Since that initial discovery, I have used the Steps of **STOP** Pain, in combination with minimal medication, to control pain during medical procedures and after knee surgery.

You too can STOP mild to moderate pain and reduce severe or chronic pain.

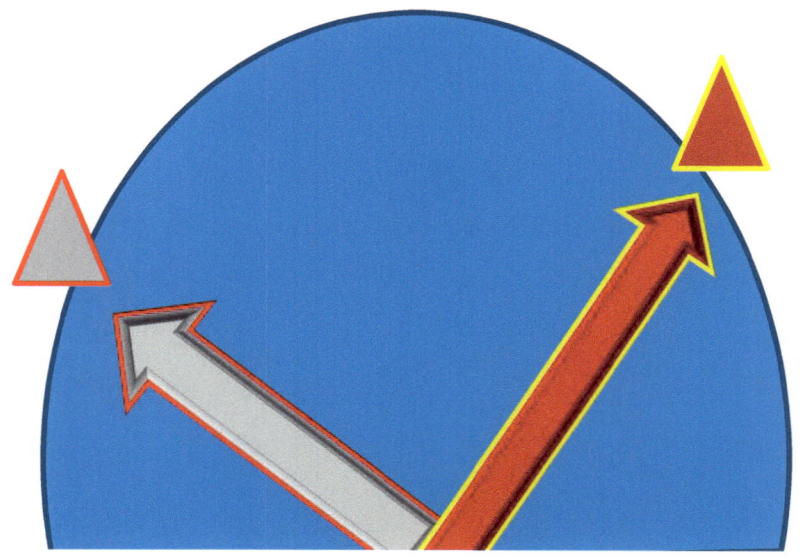

Steps of **STOP Pain**
that can help you relax,
turn your attention
away from pain and
empower yourself.

Steps of
STOP Pain

Slowly breathe.

Tune-out & picture
a peaceful place.

Open your imagination
to add action & music.

Positively "self-direct."
(Tell yourself to relax
and be calm)

1) **S**lowly breathe.

Slow deep breathing calms emotions and cools pain.

Pain triggers the "fight or flight" response of our emotional system, which is deep in the brain. It is much like a submarine deep under the ocean. The best way we can communicate with it is by sending the "calming signal" of slow and deep breathing.

2) **T**une-out & picture a peaceful place.

Turn your attention

away from pain,

as you tune-out from the

"pain broadcasting center."

&

picture a peaceful place

to trigger the

relaxation response.

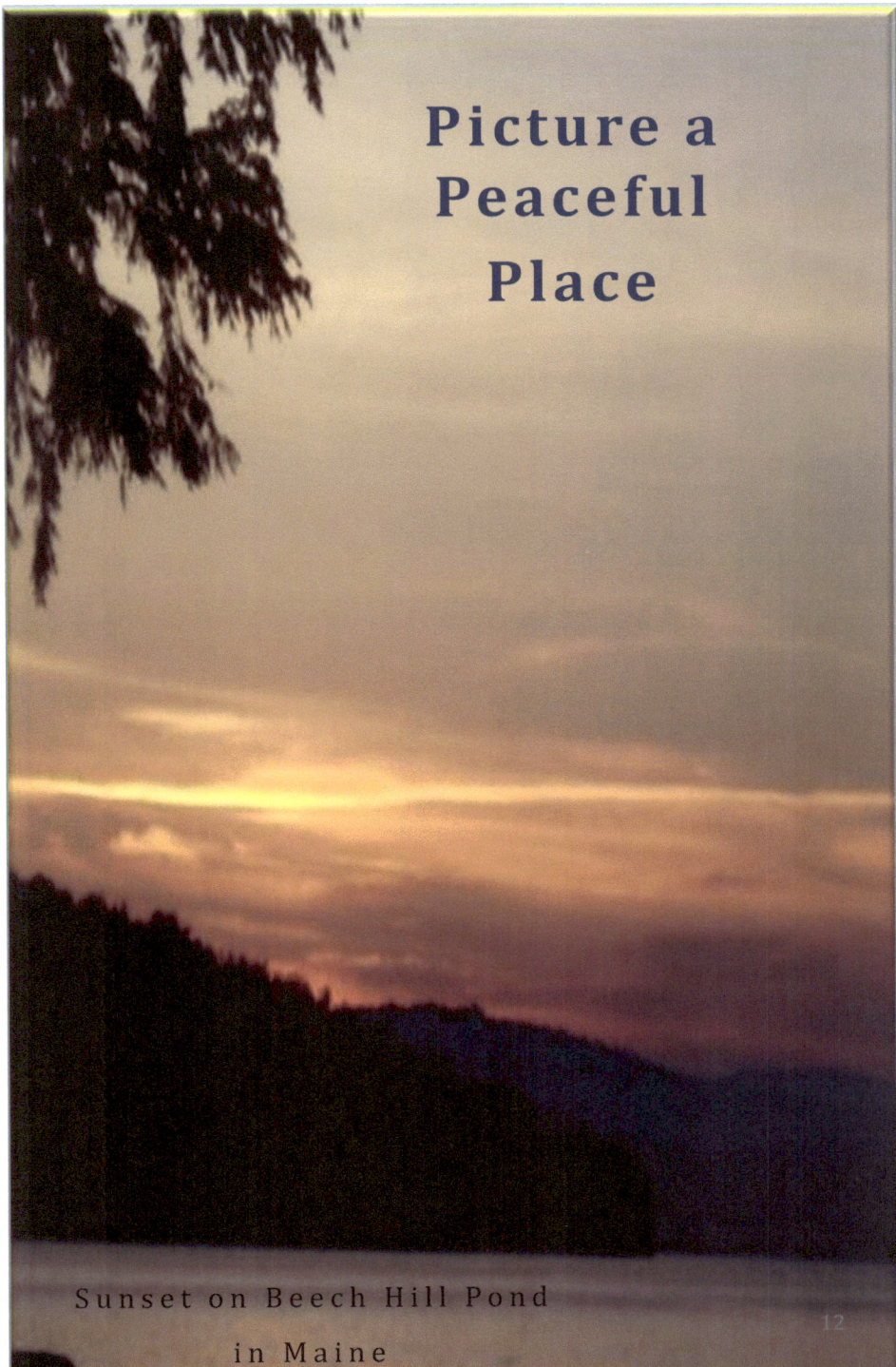

Picture a Peaceful Place

Sunset on Beech Hill Pond in Maine

3) **O**pen your imagination to add action & music.

Open your imagination to **add action** to the scene you are imagining.

For example, imagine clouds floating by or birds flying across a sunset.

Then, play pleasant **music in your mind** from your "musical memory collection."

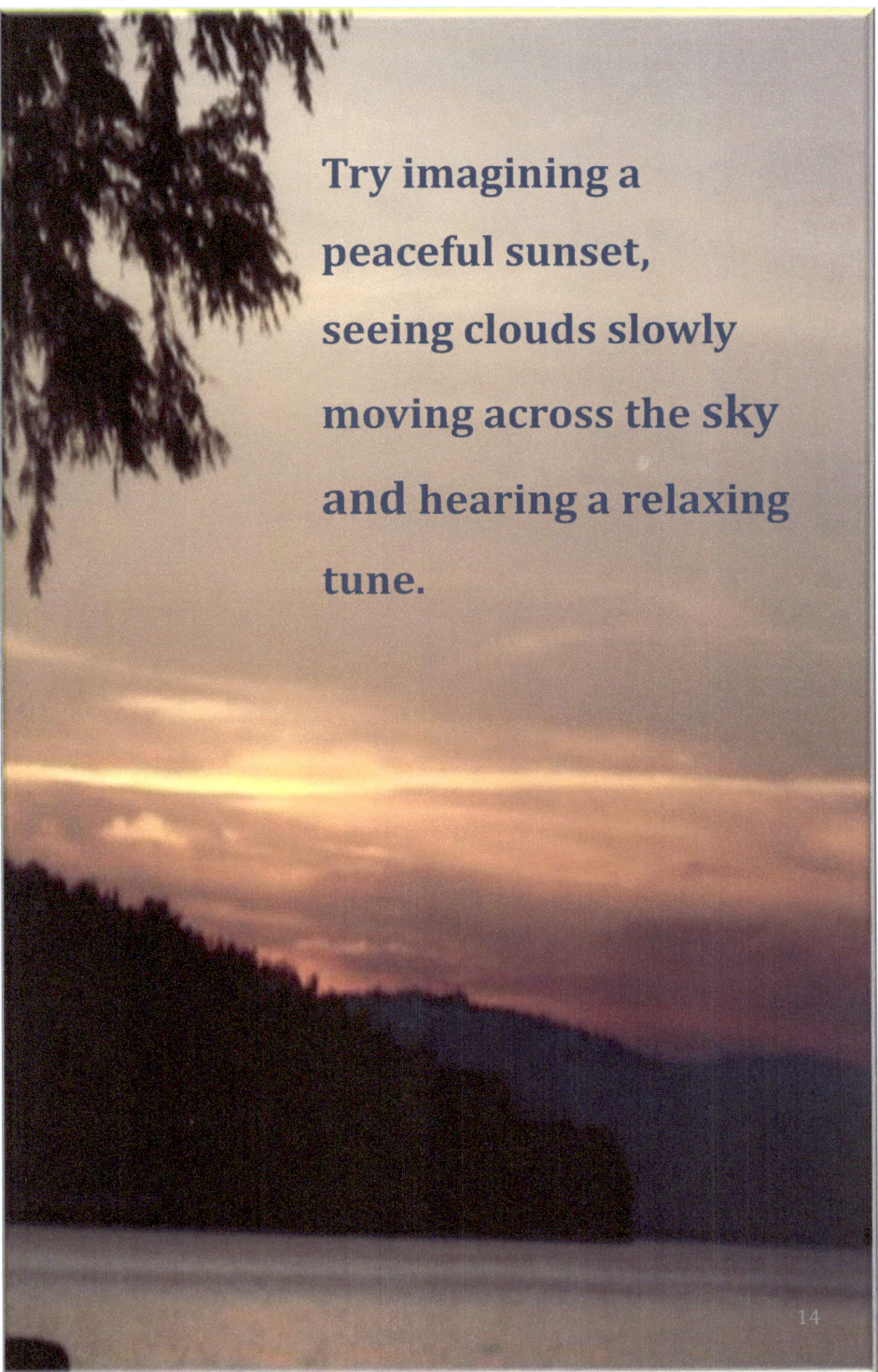

Try imagining a peaceful sunset, seeing clouds slowly moving across the sky and hearing a relaxing tune.

4) **P**ositively "self-direct."

To help your body relax, positively "self-direct" by talking to yourself in your own mind.

For example, tell yourself,
**"I'm going to relax.
I'm just going to let
my whole body relax
and be calm."**

Steps of

STOP Pain

can be the first line

of defense

against pain!

Practice the Steps of STOP Pain to perfect the skill

Regular practice
of the Steps of **STOP** Pain
trains your body and helps make
self-calming more automatic.
Repeated practice perfects most skills,
much as it does in athletics
or playing musical instruments.
Think of your body as a musical
instrument that requires practice
to be able to play a mellow tune.

Also, consider using repeated practice
of the Steps of **STOP**
as a kind of daily meditation.

Medication may also be needed for more severe or persistent pain.

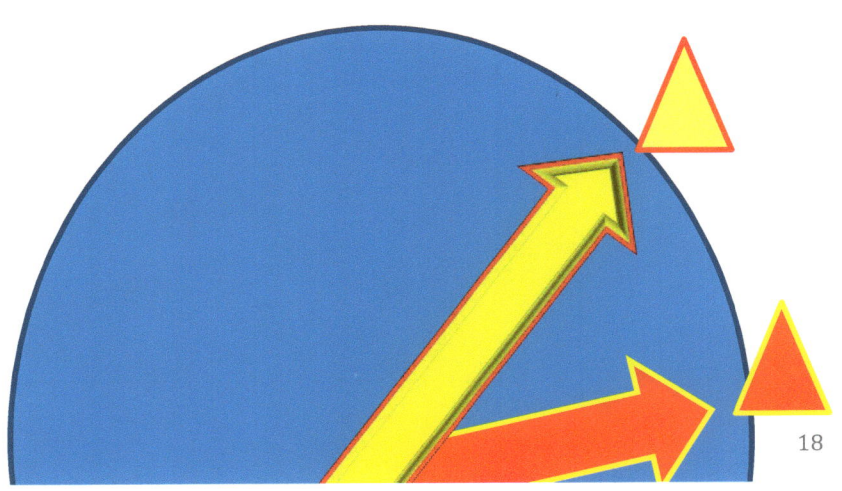

However, use medication very cautiously!

Even non-prescription pain medication can be harmful when used excessively.

For example, "Ibuprofen" can damage the kidneys and "Tylenol" can damage the liver when used excessively.

**Narcotic
pain medication
can become
very addictive
when too much
is used,
or for too long.**

**Therefore, narcotic
pain medication
should be used only when
needed, very sparingly
and for a limited time!**

On the other hand,

the steps of **STOP** Pain

can team-up with medication

to reduce the amount of

medication needed

to control pain.

Then, the steps of

STOP Pain

can help relieve pain,

while reducing medication's

risk of harm or addiction.

Comparisons between medication and the steps of STOP Pain

- **Medication has a delayed effect.**

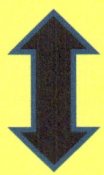

- **The steps of STOP Pain work immediately.**

Comparisons continued:

➢ The delayed effect of medication encourages early use of pain medication to avoid pain before it begins.
**Repeated early use
of medication to avoid pain can
lead to addiction**.

➢ The steps of **STOP Pain** can help control any pain that **might** occur while waiting for medication to work, thus preventing the need for avoidant use of medication.

To Stop addiction,
**"An ounce of prevention
is worth a pound of cure**!"

Comparisons continued:

➢ When medication is used to avoid pain, the fear of pain may grow, and increasing fear of pain can feed harmful addictions!

(<u>Explanation</u>: Fear of pain generates anxiety, which is reduced when medication is taken to avoid pain. Anxiety reduction is a very powerful reward that reinforces and empowers the fear of pain, thus creating a "vicious cycle.")

➢ The Steps of **STOP** Pain can reduce both pain and the fear of pain. Repeated use of the Steps of **STOP** Pain can lead to a "beneficial cycle," since it reduces stress and increases a general feeling of well-being.

Comparisons continued:

➤ Fear of a painful medical procedure can increase the amount of medication needed to control pain during the procedure.

➤ The steps of STOP Pain can be used to relax before a painful procedure begins and reduce the amount of medication needed to control pain during the procedure.

Comparisons continued

➢ Because the body habituates to narcotic medication, it can become less effective the more you use it, which can lead to an increasing need for narcotic medication to control pain.

➢ The steps of **STOP Pain** use the body's "Natural Power," which becomes more effective the more you use it, in a self-empowering cycle.

Comparisons continued:

➤ **Pain can keep you captive!**

➤ **The steps of STOP Pain can help free you from pain!**

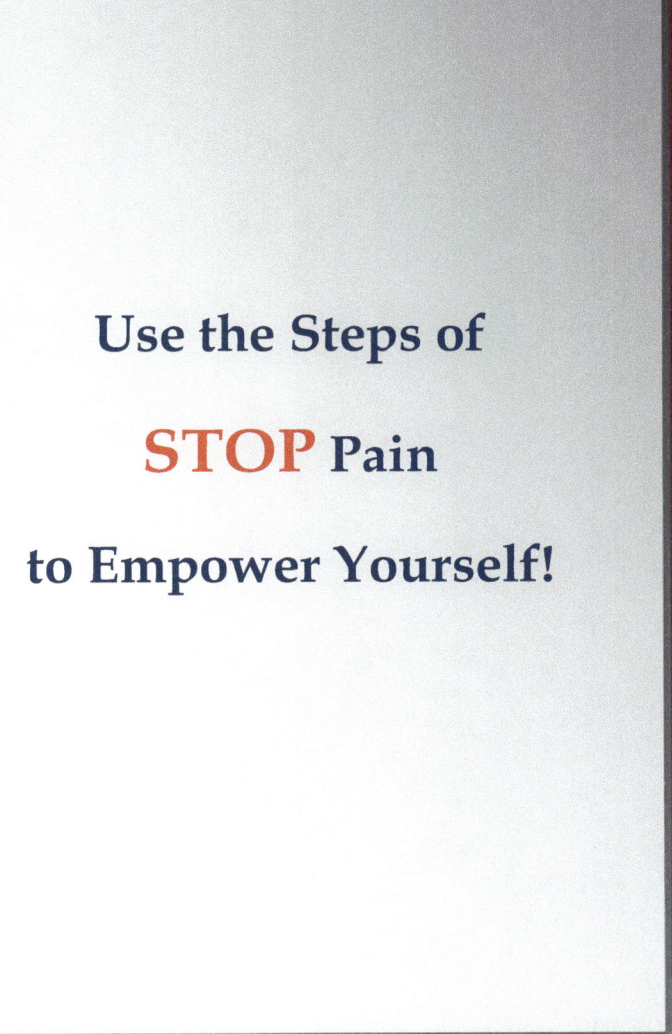

Use the Steps of

STOP Pain

to Empower Yourself!

Practice the Steps
of **STOP**

Slowly breathe.

Tune-out & imagine
a peaceful place.

Open your imagination
to action &. Music.

Positively self-direct
by telling yourself
to relax & be calm.

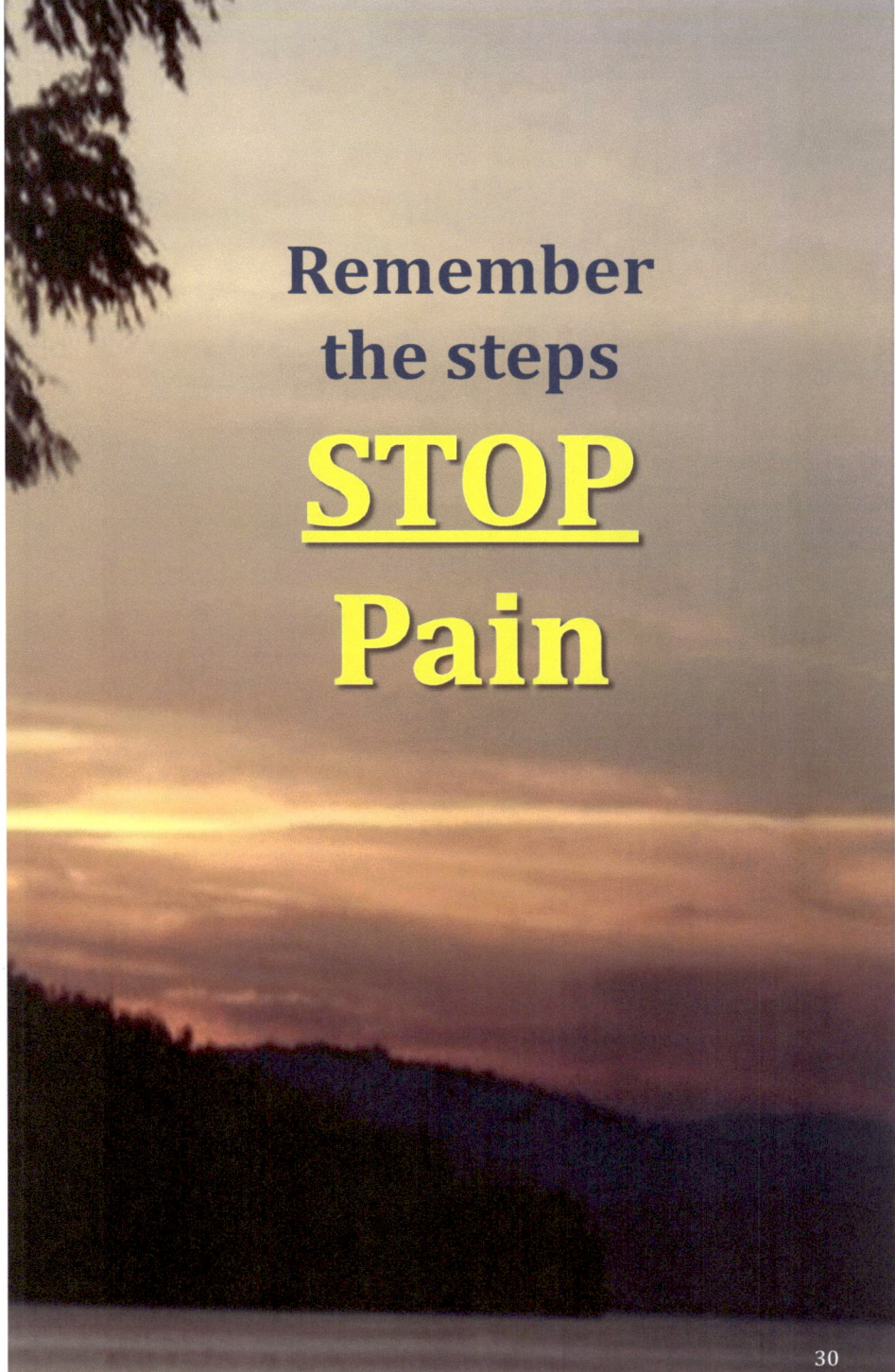

To **STOP** P a i n, remember to:

Slowly breathe.

Tune-out & picture a peaceful place.

Open your imagination to music & action.

Positively "self-direct" (tell yourself to relax and be calm.)

A version of the steps of STOP can also help you relax and go to sleep.

STOP to relax & go to sleep at night.

Slowly breathe.

Tune-out and picture a peaceful place.

Open your imagination to add music and action.

Positively "self-direct" by telling yourself: "I'm getting sleepier, and sleepier, and sleep, sleep-- sleep -– slee ----- slee -------- "

Use of Steps of STOP Pain on Mobile Phones and Tablets.

Go to *Amazon.com* and download the Kindle App for your mobile phone or tablet.

<u>How to best use steps as self-cues to gain power over pain</u>

1) Read descriptions steps of STOP Pain to understand how they work.

2) Practice steps to perfect self-calming.

3) Use the steps of **STOP Pain** to gain power over pain.

About the Author

Dr. Bob Peddicord is a Clinical Psychologist. He developed the steps of **STOP** Pain to help manage pain.

He has also taught the Steps of **STOP** Pain to numerous clients to help them deal with fears, panic, and other painful emotions.

To see other publications by Dr. Bob, please go to **Amazon.com** and search for Dr. Bob Peddicord

Thanks to Clyde Comstock
for his fantastic "Farewell" photograph

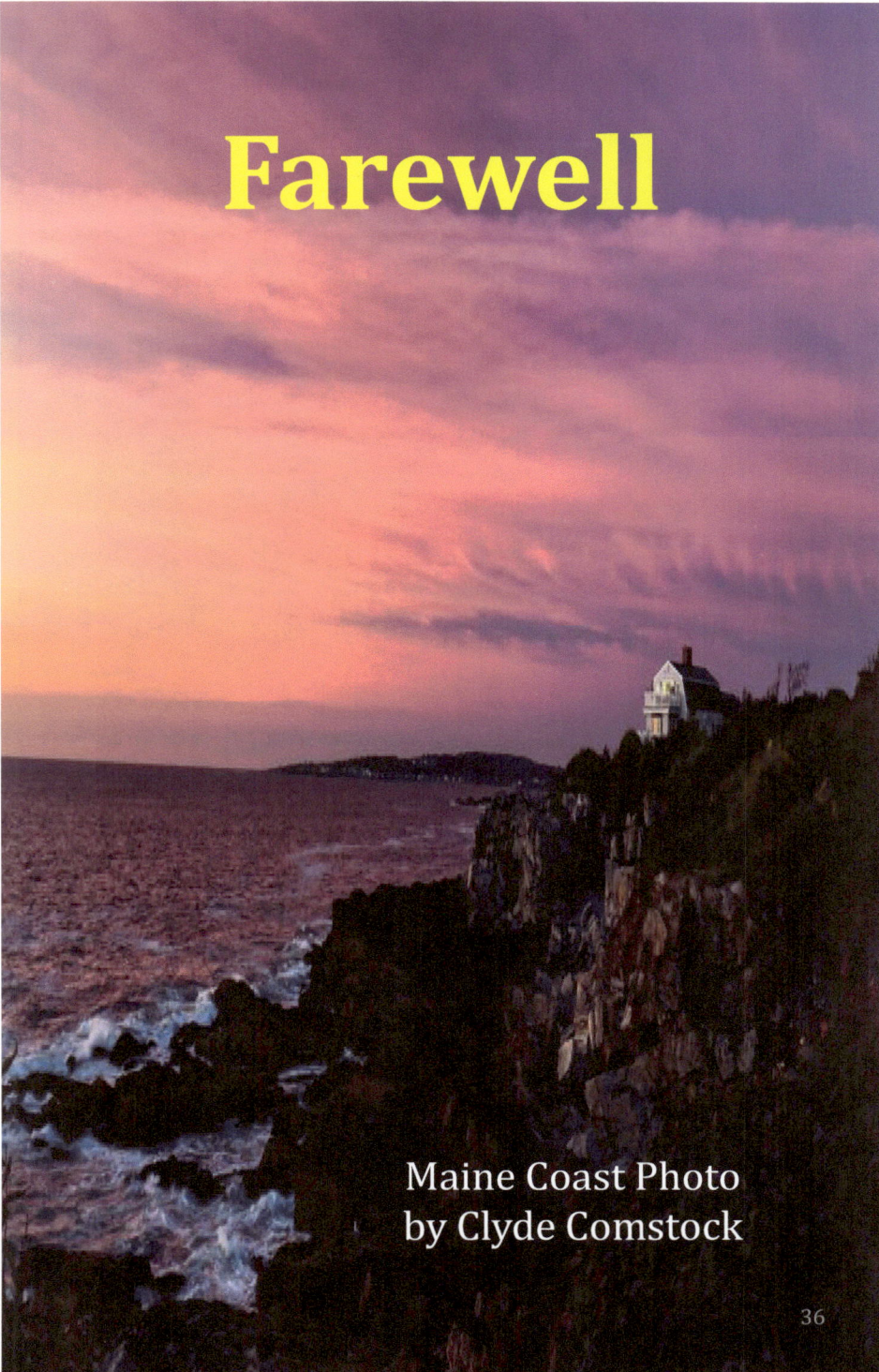

Farewell

Maine Coast Photo
by Clyde Comstock

Steps of
STOP Pain

Slowly breathe.

Tune-out & picture a peaceful place.

Open your imagination to music & action.

Positively "self-direct."
(Tell yourself to relax and be calm)

www.ingramcontent.com/pod-product-compliance
Lightning Source LLC
Chambersburg PA
CBHW040254220526
45473CB00001B/478